FACILITATOR GUIDE

ETHICAL CASE STUDIES FOR ADVANCED PRACTICE NURSES

Solving Dilemmas in Everyday Practice

Amber L. Vermeesch, PhD, MSN, RN, FNP-C, FACSM, FNAP, ANEF

Patricia H. Cox, DNP, MPH, MN, BSN, RN

Inga M. Giske, DNP, MSN, RN, PMHNP-BC, PMH-BC, NE-BC

Katherine M. Roberts, DNP, BSN, RN, FNP-C

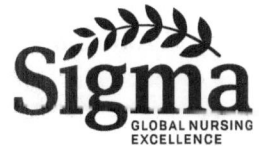

Copyright © 2023 by Sigma Theta Tau International Honor Society of Nursing

All rights reserved. This book is protected by copyright. No part of it may be reproduced, stored in a retrieval system, or transmitted in any form or by any means, electronic, mechanical, photocopying, recording, or otherwise, without written permission from the publisher. Any trademarks, service marks, design rights, or similar rights that are mentioned, used, or cited in this book are the property of their respective owners. Their use here does not imply that you may use them for a similar or any other purpose.

This book is not intended to be a substitute for the medical advice of a licensed medical professional. The author and publisher have made every effort to ensure the accuracy of the information contained within at the time of its publication and shall have no liability or responsibility to any person or entity regarding any loss or damage incurred, or alleged to have incurred, directly or indirectly, by the information contained in this book. The author and publisher make no warranties, express or implied, with respect to its content, and no warranties may be created or extended by sales representatives or written sales materials. The author and publisher have no responsibility for the consistency or accuracy of URLs and content of third-party websites referenced in this book.

Sigma Theta Tau International Honor Society of Nursing (Sigma) is a nonprofit organization whose mission is developing nurse leaders anywhere to improve healthcare everywhere. Founded in 1922, Sigma has more than 135,000 active members in over 100 countries and territories. Members include practicing nurses, instructors, researchers, policymakers, entrepreneurs, and others. Sigma's more than 540 chapters are located at more than 700 institutions of higher education throughout Armenia, Australia, Botswana, Brazil, Canada, Colombia, Croatia, England, Eswatini, Ghana, Hong Kong, Ireland, Israel, Italy, Jamaica, Japan, Jordan, Kenya, Lebanon, Malawi, Mexico, the Netherlands, Nigeria, Pakistan, Philippines, Portugal, Puerto Rico, Scotland, Singapore, South Africa, South Korea, Sweden, Taiwan, Tanzania, Thailand, the United States, and Wales. Learn more at www.sigmanursing.org.

Sigma Theta Tau International
550 West North Street
Indianapolis, IN, USA 46202

To request a review copy for course adoption, order additional books, buy in bulk, or purchase for corporate use, contact Sigma Marketplace at 888.654.4968 (US/Canada toll-free), +1.317.687.2256 (International), or solutions@sigmamarketplace.org.

To request author information, or for speaker or other media requests, contact Sigma Marketing at 888.634.7575 (US/Canada toll-free) or +1.317.634.8171 (International).

PRINT ISBN: 9781646480975
PDF ISBN: 9781646480982

First Printing, 2023

Publisher: Dustin Sullivan
Acquisitions Editor: Emily Hatch
Development Editor: Jillmarie Leeper Sycamore
Cover Designer: Rebecca Batchelor
Interior Design/Page Layout: Rebecca Batchelor

Managing Editor: Carla Hall
Publications Specialist: Todd Lothery
Project Editor: Jillmarie Leeper Sycamore
Copy Editor: Todd Lothery
Proofreader: Todd Lothery

About the Authors

Amber L. Vermeesch, PhD, MSN, RN, FNP-C, FACSM, FNAP, ANEF, has been a practicing family nurse practitioner since 2006. She has spent most of her practice serving underinsured and vulnerable populations. She completed her master's in nursing at Vanderbilt University School of Nursing. She earned her PhD in nursing science from the University of Miami in 2011, where she focused on reducing healthcare disparities among Latino populations using multiple methodologies, including participatory photography. She joined the University of Portland as an Associate Professor in 2014, teaching in both graduate and undergraduate programs, and served as the Director of Research and Scholarship. She became a certified nurse educator in 2017. In 2022, Vermeesch was inducted as a Fellow in the National League for Nursing Academy of Nursing Education; in 2020, she became a Fellow in the American College of Sports Medicine as well as Distinguished Practitioner and Fellow in the National Academies of Practice. Her overall area of expertise is wellness, both physical and emotional. In 2022, she became the Department Chair for Family and Community Nursing at the University of North Carolina at Greensboro. Her investigations have concentrated on physical activity and integrated health among vulnerable populations. Additionally, she explores risk factors related to stress reduction and health promotion among undergraduates and graduate students as well as faculty and staff. Patricia Cox (2014–2015) and Vermeesch (2015–2016) laid the initial foundations for this workbook through individual fellowship projects in the Application of Ethics provided by the Dundon-Berchtold Institute. All four main authors— Cox, Vermeesch, Inga Giske, and Katherine Roberts— participated in the Ethics Curriculum Fellowship 2019–2020 provided by the Dundon-Berchtold Institute to develop those projects into this workbook.

Patricia H. Cox, DNP, MPH, MN, BSN, RN, recently retired as the Director of Doctoral Nursing Education & Practice at the School of Nursing at the University of Portland. Her long career in nursing took her from the bedside as an Army nurse to working as a public health nurse with migrant farmworkers and then Lao refugees in Thailand. Along the way, she advanced her education while caring for HIV/AIDS patients as a nurse practitioner in the early days of the epidemic. Later she provided primary care to Native American and Hispanic populations in a community clinic in Los Angeles. Always supportive of nursing education, Cox served as adjunct faculty in several nursing programs prior to relocating to Portland to teach full time and prepare the next generation of nurse practitioners in the DNP Program at the University of Portland.

Inga M. Giske, DNP, MSN, RN, PMHNP-BC, PMH-BC, NE-BC, serves as a psychiatric nurse practitioner on the Psychiatric Consult-Liaison service at Providence St. Vincent Medical Center. She provides psychiatric evaluation and treatment recommendations for patients during their medical admission while also providing education and support to professional staff, nursing, and ancillary care team members. In addition, she serves as a preceptor to nurse practitioner students, medical students, and internal medicine residents. Her nursing career has spanned from bedside nursing to regional leadership in acute inpatient psychiatric units and psychiatric emergency departments. She implemented evidence-based practice changes in both acute inpatient and psychiatric settings to reduce falls and violence and improve patient and caregiver satisfaction. Giske works to improve knowledge regarding mental health conditions and reduce stigma through education of nurses, other healthcare providers, and her community. She has been adjunct faculty at the University of Portland, teaching undergraduate psychiatric nursing. She provides competency-based suicide assessment training to nurses both locally and nationally. Lastly, she has served as a trainer to local law enforcement in her community, educating both new recruits and experienced officers on mental health, crisis intervention, and de-escalation for the past six years.

Katherine Roberts, DNP, BSN, RN, FNP-C, is a recent DNP graduate from the University of Portland. Although new to the DNP role, she has an extensive background as a bachelor-prepared registered nurse. After graduating from Linfield College in 2004, Roberts has practiced in various settings, including the Childhood Development and Rehabilitation Center at Doernbecher Children's Hospital and Neonatal Intensive Care Unit at Randell's Children's hospital in Portland. More recently and for most of her career, she worked for Northwest Primary Care Group. Her experience with patients extends to all ages and stages of life and various levels of care, from a nursing assistant working with developmentally and physically disabled children to a bedside nurse working with well and ill newborn and preterm infants. Eventually, she found her passion in family medicine, working with patients of all ages, including pregnant women. As a nursing leader, Roberts worked as a charge nurse for many years before eventually taking a more administrative role writing policy and procedure and creating a unique nursing and patient education program. In May 2018, she lost her friend and mentor, Dr. Margret "Peggy" McNichol, who began her career as a nurse and always taught her to strive to make the world a better place, one problem and patient at a time. Thus, Roberts decided to advance her education, get back to direct patient care, and continue making a difference for the patients and profession of nursing as a doctorally prepared nurse practitioner.

Contents

About the Authors 3
Introduction 7

CASE STUDY #1
Defensive Medicine 8

CASE STUDY #2
STI Confidentiality 10

CASE STUDY #3
Substance use in Pregnancy 13

CASE STUDY #4
HPV Vaccine Refusal 16

CASE STUDY #5
Abortion 18

CASE STUDY #6
Prostate Cancer Screening With Prostate-Specific Antigen 21

CASE STUDY #7
Administration of Long-Acting Injectable Antipsychotics 23

CASE STUDY #8
Depression Screening in Adolescents 26

CASE STUDY #9
Treatment of Resistant Anxiety 30

CASE STUDY #10
COVID-19 Vaccine in
Adolescence 32

CASE STUDY #11
Medical Emancipation Versus Confidentiality in Transgender and
Gender-Nonconforming People 34

CASE STUDY #12
Childhood Obesity 37

CASE STUDY #13
Dementia and Stopping Driving 39

CASE STUDY #14
When to Transition to Palliative Care 42

CASE STUDY #15
Prescription Refill Dilemma for Patient and Spouse in Financial Straits.................................44

CASE STUDY #16
CRNA Labor and Delivery Epidural Pain Management With a Language Barrier 46

CASE STUDY #17
Violence, Suicide, and Family Dynamics With Medical Complexity 49

CASE STUDY #18
Psychiatric Acute Concerns and Fall Risks 55

CASE STUDY #19
Telehealth 58

CASE STUDY #20
Guiding a School of Nursing Through COVID-19 Focusing on Clinical Placements............64

CASE STUDY #21
Emergency Department Closure Decision-Making: Health System and
Community Impact..66

CASE STUDY #22
Ethical Dilemmas in School of Nursing Leadership Pre-COVID-19 69

Introduction

Ethics seems to make both students and faculty nervous—a question of whether we know enough or truly understand it. We hope this Facilitator Guide—a companion to our textbook, *Ethical Case Studies for Advanced Practice Nurses*—will help you see the utility of using a framework and become more comfortable in working through the ethical dilemmas presented to come to a resolution. The steps to using the framework are clearly laid out in each chapter of the book after the case study is presented. This guide provides additional questions to assist in facilitating discussion in the classroom.

Prior to class, students can read the case study and be prepared to respond to each of the steps. The case studies are from real-life situations that require thoughtful critical analysis. Each discussion should represent current practice, policies, and laws in your individual state or organization.

Thank you for choosing our textbook to aid you in discussing ethical dilemmas for advanced practice nursing students.

We wish you fortitude and wisdom in creating and providing solutions for your ethical dilemmas.

Drs. Vermeesch, Cox, Giske, and Roberts

"Let whoever is in charge keep this simple question in her head (not, how can I always do this right thing myself, but) how can I provide for this right thing to be always done?"

—Florence Nightingale

CASE STUDY #1

DEFENSIVE MEDICINE

This case study represents a frequent occurrence for primary care nurse practitioner students and new nurse practitioner providers: how to provide competent and safe care in a litigious healthcare environment.

Consider:

1. Identify the ethical concerns with this situation.

    - Is the dilemma to provide appropriate care to the patient or to protect the provider? Or both?

    - What are the potential implications of doing unnecessary testing, thinking of both the patient and the healthcare system?

2. What information will you need before a responsible decision can be made? (Consider what the information is and where it will come from.)

    - Are there guidelines available to assist you in providing care to this patient? What is the patient's expectation?

    - What is the prevalence of the disease in the community?

    - What does the history and physical exam reveal about the patient's condition?

3. Who are the stakeholders involved in the decision, and what is the process in which those involved could come to a decision (e.g., what tools are/could be used to create an informed decision)?

   - The patient: What does the patient think is the problem? Have you included them in the discussion?

   - The provider: Does the patient's insurance cover the diagnostic test? What are the patient's financial resources if insurance does not cover additional testing or the patient has a large deductible? Is the provider following the clinical guidelines? Is the provider following the organization's policies?

   - The healthcare system: Would further testing make a difference in the care plan?

4. What are the values relevant to this problem? *Values* are the things that you believe are important in making the decision. They (should) determine priorities. Values relevant to this problem may not be representative of your own personal values or moral framework.

   - With unnecessary testing or lack of testing, what harm could come to the patient and to the practice?

   - What would be the benefit to the patient and/or practice?

   - Consider solidarity, integrity, and patient welfare.

5. What are the options for the decision? Think in terms of values and feasibility (e.g., financial, political, organizational, religious constraints).

   - Should everything be done?

   - Should nothing be done?

   - Should some testing be done but not others? If so, which will give you the information that will likely inform your plan of care?

Management of Case Study

After all considerations, write a short narrative describing the best way to manage this situation; list core values important to you for managing it.

CASE STUDY #2

STI CONFIDENTIALITY

Confidentiality is of the utmost importance when serving patients in healthcare. It allows patients freedom to confide in the provider and feel safe from persecution by others. However, it is incredibly important that the advanced practice nurse understand when confidentiality must be secondary to ensuring patient care and safety.

Consider:

1. Identify the ethical concerns with this situation.

    - Are there ways to ensure safety and proper care for the patient and the patient's husband?

    - If the patient's husband were to find out about his wife's infidelity, could there be consequences for the nurse practitioner and the patient?

    - What harm could come if all parties are not appropriately treated?

2. What information will you need before a responsible decision can be made? (Consider what the information is and where it will come from.)

    - Is the patient's husband at risk for long-term effects?

    - What is the state reporting law/requirement for infectious diseases? Where can you find it?

    - Knowing the law, consider what is mandated for the advanced practice nurse and what is not.

    - Are there guidelines that assist a provider in their "duty to warn"? Where can these be found?

3. Who are the stakeholders involved in the decision, and what is the process in which those involved could come to a decision (e.g., what tools are/could be used to create an informed decision)?

   - Provider: Will you report the patient's STI and her partner?

   - Patient: Wouldn't the patient want to know she was exposed if it were her husband who had an STI?

   - Patient's partners: Should the patient disclose to her young male partner that she has sought care for her STI?

   - Public health department: What tools does the department offer to have difficult conversations with patients about STIs?

   - Law enforcement: What tools are provided by law enforcement to prevent domestic violence?

4. Are there other providers or specialists to consult that have experience with similar scenarios? Are there educational materials you can review?

   - State or local public health office

   - CDC STI treatment guidelines

   - Infectious disease specialist

   - Women's health provider

   - Personal colleague

   - UpToDate

   - Nursing/medical journals

5. Are there safeguards to protect the patient if abuse is occurring in the home?

   - Organization social worker

   - State or local social services

   - State or local department of family/human services

6. What are the values relevant to this problem? *Values* are the things that you believe are important in making the decision. They (should) determine priorities. Values relevant to this problem may not be representative of your own personal values or moral framework.

   - What is the provider's responsibility—to inform the public health department or not? Does state law play a role here?

   - What are the patient's rights in this situation?

- How can you reassure the patient that reporting the STI and informing her husband is needed?
- Can you assist the patient with the language to use to inform her partners on her own?

7. What are the options for the decision? Think in terms of values and feasibility (e.g., financial, political, organizational, religious constraints).

- Does the provider have an obligation to only the patient or to her husband too?
- Does suspected abuse play a role in the decision and options that are available?
- Are there consequences if the patient does not inform her husband and the provider does not inform the county health department? What may these consequences be, and do they play a role in the decision?

Management of Case Study

After all considerations, write a short narrative describing the best way to manage this situation; list core values important to you for managing the situation.

CASE STUDY #3

SUBSTANCE USE IN PREGNANCY

Substance use disorder in pregnancy affects both the woman and unborn fetus. Advanced practice providers must put aside personal opinions and values to care for both the patient and the fetus, regardless of how challenging it may be. In certain places women are forced into punitive treatment programs or are legally penalized for substance use in pregnancy, making it less likely for a woman to seek proper prenatal care or alternatively seek abortion services.

Consider:

1. Identify the ethical concerns with this situation.

    - Knowing that the patient prefers not to see a physician, what are the options, considering the patient's right to autonomy?

    - How can the advanced practice nurse ensure that civil liberty and justice are taken into consideration? Should the advanced practice nurse treat this patient as any other pregnant person, or are there other aspects to consider?

    - If the mother does not seek further treatment with someone that has experience caring for mothers with substance use disorders, are there implications concerning beneficence and non-maleficence for both the mother and child? Examples: physical harm to both mother and fetus, psychosocial harm to mother.

2. What information will you need before a responsible decision can be made? (Consider what the information is and where it will come from.)

    - Is the pregnancy desired?

    - Is there a willingness to reduce or quit the substance?

    - What kind of substance is involved, and what are the possible implications for the patient and the fetus?

- What are the resources to find this information? Examples: American College of Obstetricians and Gynecologists, UpToDate.

- Are there options for treatment programs? What are they? Is the patient willing to participate in treatment if it is available?

- As a provider, what is your responsibility to the patient and to the unborn fetus? Where can you find this information? Example: Substance Abuse and Mental Health Services Administration (SAMHSA).

3. Who are the stakeholders involved in the decision, and what is the process in which those involved could come to a decision (e.g., what tools are/could be used to create an informed decision)?

    - Patient: What does the patient need for a successful pregnancy?

    - Provider: How can the advanced practice provider build trust with the patient? What role does trust play in making an informed decision? How can the advanced practice registered nurse assist the patient in getting the care she and her unborn fetus need? What resources are available?
        - Centers for Disease Control and Prevention
        - SAMHSA
        - Local/county health department

    - Specialists: What specialist would you refer the patient to?

    - Treatment programs: What programs are available in your area?

    - Child welfare/social services: Do you need to refer your patient to child welfare services?

4. What are the values relevant to this problem? *Values* are the things that you believe are important in making the decision. They (should) determine priorities. Values relevant to this problem may not be representative of your own personal values or moral framework.

    - What is the provider's responsibility to both the patient and the unborn fetus? Does the patient require specialty care?

    - What types of treatment does this patient need, and does the patient consent to recommended treatment? What if she does not consent?

    - What would be the best way to build trust in this situation, as the patient has had a poor experience with healthcare in the past?

    - Should you allow the patient to decide on a treatment program? Are there non-punitive treatment programs available?

    - Does the patient have the means and support needed for herself and unborn fetus?

    - If substance use disorder is considered a disease, what comfort and difficulty measures must be considered for the patient to ensure that the fetus is safe?

5. What are the options for the decision? Think in terms of values and feasibility (e.g., financial, political, organizational, religious constraints).

    - Does the patient have the means to seek treatment, both financially and considering time off from work?

    - Does anyone need to be notified about the unborn fetus being at risk?

    - Are there resources available to assist in making an informed decision?

    - Are there specialists that could be consulted?

    - Is caring for the patient outside of the APRN's scope? Would there be a time when this may be appropriate or not?

Management of Case Study

After all considerations, write a short narrative describing the best way to manage this situation; list core values important to you for managing the situation.

CASE STUDY #4

HPV VACCINE REFUSAL

The human papillomavirus (HPV) vaccination has been proven effective to protect against various forms of the HPV virus. However, regardless of the evidence, there are shockingly low rates of vaccination among teenagers, who make up the demographic recommended to receive the vaccine. Literature shows that parents find the vaccination to be unnecessary if their children are "not sexually active" and feel that if the vaccine is administered it may lead to risky sexual behavior.

Consider:

1. Identify the ethical concerns with this situation.

   - Because the patient is a boy and is at less risk of developing complications of HPV, should he be excluded from getting the vaccine?

   - Are others at risk if the patient becomes sexually active and he remains unvaccinated? If so, who?

   - Are the concerns of the mother valid? What could the advanced practice nurse do for the mother and the patient to build trust? What information will you need before a responsible decision can be made? (Consider what the information is and where it will come from.)

   - What is the mother's health literacy, and how did she come to the conclusions about the vaccine that she has?

   - Is the patient aware of the purpose of the vaccine? Could informing him help with the decision?

   - What is the advanced practice nurse's role in the discussion? Is it to persuade or inform?

2. Who are the stakeholders involved in the decision, and what is the process in which those involved could come to a decision (e.g., what tools are/could be used to create an informed decision)?

    - Patient: How can you best support Ethan?

    - Patient's mother: What additional education can you provide the mother? Would motivational interviewing help?

    - Advanced practice nurse: What is the best way to inform the mother of the benefits of the vaccine? For example, the Centers for Disease Control and Prevention website, vaccine information statements, the World Health Organization website? What other shared decision-making materials are available to you?

3. What are the values relevant to this problem? *Values* are the things that you believe are important in making the decision. They (should) determine priorities. Values relevant to this problem may not be representative of your own personal values or moral framework.

    - How do you advocate for the patient and future partners?

    - How do you educate the mother and reassure the patient and continue to build trust? Do the patient and parent trust the advanced practice nurse?

    - How do you support the decisions made by the patient and mother?

4. What are the options for the decision? Think in terms of values and feasibility (e.g., financial, political, organizational, religious constraints).

    - Do the patient and parent have the health literacy and information required about the vaccine?

    - Are there religious barriers that the advanced practice nurse should be aware of?

    - Could the advanced practice nurse try and persuade the patient and his parent?

    - Could the advanced practice nurse not engage with the mother knowing she will not change her mind?

Management of Case Study

After all considerations, write a short narrative describing the best way to manage this situation; list core values important to you for managing the situation.

CASE STUDY #5

ABORTION

At one time, access to medical abortion influenced a substantial decline in maternal mortality and morbidity. However, some medical professionals have found themselves in a moral conundrum when it comes to the practice of abortion. Furthermore, since the Supreme Court's overturning of Roe v. Wade, medical abortions are illegal in many states. Thus, it is important for the advanced practice nurse to be aware of the laws where they practice and have a firm grasp of ethically sound ways to assist a patient with what they want and need.

Consider:

1. Identify the ethical concerns with this situation.

- What if the advanced practice nurse were to withhold abortion information or treatment that the patient desires because of their own moral code?

- Should autonomy for the patient's wishes to terminate the pregnancy play a role, even though there is an unborn fetus involved?

- Although abortion is legal in the state of Oregon, is it right to do if a woman's or unborn fetus' health is not at risk?

- Should a woman have the right to choose what she does with her own body such as terminate a pregnancy that she does not desire?

- Has the patient's partner been notified, and should he have a say on whether to terminate the unborn fetus?

- Could the advanced practice nurse's morals and position of authority change the patient's mind? If so, would this be ethically sound?

- Could a medical abortion cause health concerns for the patient during the procedure or in the future?

2. What information will you need before a responsible decision can be made? (Consider what the information is and where it will come from.)

    - Does the patient have all the necessary information needed to make an informed decision?

    - Does the patient understand the implications of a medical abortion and how her body will respond?

    - Is the patient of sound mind to make the decision to terminate her pregnancy?

    - Does the law allow for abortions to be done legally, and where would this information be found?

    - Would there be any repercussions to the patient or provider if the advanced practice nurse prescribed a medical abortion? (Think both legally and morally.)

    - Are there other choices besides abortion that the patient has not thought about?

    - How will having a child affect the patient's future?

    - Could stigma of being unwed and young be a deciding factor for the patient? How does this play into making an informed decision?

    - Are there any other options for the advanced practice nurse to help the patient without attempting to persuade the patient against abortion?

3. Who are the stakeholders involved in the decision, and what is the process in which those involved could come to a decision (e.g., what tools are/could be used to create an informed decision)?

    - Patient: Is she educated enough about the procedure? If not, what could be provided to ensure that the patient is informed? Does the patient have the means to get a medical abortion?

    - Fathering partner: Does he need to be considered?

    - Advanced practice nurse: What information does she need to assist the patient?

    - Provider's organization: Do they allow providers to practice medical abortions?

    - Colleagues of the advanced practice nurse: Do any colleagues have experience in providing medical abortions?

    - Specialist: Are any specialists required?

    - Patient's insurance provider: Does the patient's insurance cover medical abortions? How might one find the answer?

    - State governing body: All states have tools to locate the laws about abortion rights that vary from state to state. Do you know where to find these laws for your state?

4. What are the values relevant to this problem? *Values* are the things that you believe are important in making the decision. They (should) determine priorities. Values relevant to this problem may not be representative of your own personal values or moral framework.

   - Is the advanced practice nurse able to put aside their values and morals and either provide the medical abortion or find another way to assist the patient? What would that look like?

   - How can the advanced practice nurse ensure that the patient is able to make her own decisions regarding her health and body? (Do not forget about mental health in the situation.)

   - Does the patient and the provider have all the information they need to make an informed decision? If not, where might they find it?
     - UpToDate
     - American College of Obstetricians and Gynecologists (ACOG)

   - Does the patient have the financial means to have a medical abortion? If the provider is unable to provide care and will need to refer, does the patient have an option to seek care elsewhere?

   - Since the provider has not performed or does not have experience with this kind of care, would it be safe for the provider to provide a medical abortion?

5. What are the options for the decision? Think in terms of values and feasibility (e.g., financial, political, organizational, religious constraints).

   - Does the facility where the advanced practice nurse works allow medical abortions?

   - If the advanced practice nurse is unable to provide a medical abortion for personal or educational reasons, what are the other options?
     - Providers often will refer to someone in or outside of their organization. Is there someone internally who feels comfortable and capable with providing a medical abortion for your patient?

   - Is the patient able to pay for a medical abortion?
     - Often, insurance companies do not cover abortions, especially those with a religious affiliation.
     - What financial options are available if the patient is unable to pay?

Management of Case Study

After all considerations, write a short narrative describing the best way to manage this situation; list core values important to you for managing the situation.

Facilitator: Consider discussing a scenario where an abortion is requested in a state where it is illegal. How may the students or staff manage this scenario differently?

CASE STUDY #6

PROSTATE CANCER SCREENING WITH PROSTATE-SPECIFIC ANTIGEN

Historically, prostate cancer screening has been recommended as a universal screening for all men age 50 and older. However, since 2012, guidelines have changed, and the US Preventative Services Task Force (USPSTF) now advises against universal screening because of over diagnosing and treating for false positives. Recommendations for screening at the time of this writing are based on shared decision-making between the provider and patient. A conclusion about whether to screen should be made based on the patient's risk factors, such as family history of prostate cancer or worsening urological symptoms.

Consider:

1. Identify the ethical concerns with this situation.

    - Should the advanced practice nurse order the PSA without further conversations with the patient because her colleague told her to? Would this affect the ideals of beneficence and non-maleficence?

    - Should the advanced practice nurse decline to schedule the PSA altogether, as this is what is likely best for the patient?

2. What information will you need before a responsible decision can be made? (Consider what the information is and where it will come from.)

    - What are the current guidelines for PSA screening, and where can you find them?

    - Does the patient understand what the screening is?

    - What are the risks and benefits of having a PSA screening?

3. Who are the stakeholders involved in the decision, and what is the process in which those involved could come to a decision (e.g., what tools are/could be used to create an informed decision)?

   - Patient: Does he understand the risks and benefits?

   - Advanced practice nurse: What information does the GNP need to counsel the patient and to have the conversation with her physician colleague? Would a follow-up appointment or phone conversation be helpful in coming to a decision?

   - Physician colleague: What is the best way to educate him?

   - Patient's insurance company: Will they pay for an annual PSA?

   - The USPSTF: Do the guidelines support the decision?

4. What are the values relevant to this problem? *Values* are the things that you believe are important in making the decision. They (should) determine priorities. Values relevant to this problem may not be representative of your own personal values or moral framework.

   - Can the patient make an informed decision about his healthcare needs, and is he allowed the opportunity to do what is the best option for his health and body?

   - Is checking the PSA going to directly harm the patient? Could checking the PSA have unwanted consequences? Is checking the PSA in the best interest of the patient?

   - Can the patient trust the advanced practice nurse to have the most current guidelines? Depending on the advanced practice nurse's decision, is the patient able to trust the provider? What could the advanced practice nurse do to ensure trust and honesty?

5. What are the options for the decision? Think in terms of values and feasibility (e.g., financial, political, organizational, religious constraints).

   - Order the PSA screening?

   - Depending on shared decision-making, order the PSA screening after having a conversation with the patient about the risks and benefits?

   - Do not order the PSA screening because it is likely not in the best interest of the patient?

Management of Case Study

After all considerations, write a short narrative describing the best way to manage this situation; list core values important to you for managing the situation.

CASE STUDY #7

ADMINISTRATION OF LONG-ACTING INJECTABLE ANTIPSYCHOTICS

Due to the nationwide shortage of psychiatric providers, especially in rural areas, individuals with psychiatric disorders often face lengthy waits to access specialty care or are unable to access specialty care completely. This can result in primary care providers being asked to care for individuals in their practice whom they typically would not serve due to the inability of the person to receive services from psychiatric providers.

Consider:

1. Identify the ethical concerns with this situation.

- Does the patient demonstrate capacity to consent to the medication? If not, should he be given long-acting injectable (LAI) antipsychotics?

- Is he being coerced into treatment he does not fully understand or desire?

- Can care provided by a provider outside of their area of specialization lead to suboptimal care and outcomes for the patient and potentially harm him?

- Is some care with access to medications for treatment of bipolar disorder better than no care?

- Does it further enable the perpetuation of a broken system by giving the illusion that individuals are receiving appropriate care?

- Is this case representative of "complicated or severe mental illness" that would fall outside the scope of an FNP (Balestra, 2019)?

- How does one decide what is complicated or severe mental illness? Is it based on diagnosis, severity of symptoms, how long the patient has been stable for, the level of support they have?

2. What information will you need before a responsible decision can be made? (Consider what the information is and where it will come from.)

   - What is the patient's capacity to make an informed decision regarding the recommendation to accept the LAI antipsychotic? Capacity determinations can be made by any licensed independent provider (LIP) and must take into account the patient's ability to:
     - Express a choice
     - Understand the relevant information provided by the LIP
     - Appreciate the situation and its consequences (i.e., risks/benefits of recommended treatment/intervention)
     - Engage in rational reasoning regarding the information provided
   - Is the patient's choice being made under undue influence (Applebaum, 2007)?
   - What are the standard definitions for "complicated or severe mental illness"?
   - What are the standards for prescribing LAI medications?
   - What resources are available to the LIP such as psychiatric consultation or telepsych?

3. Who are the stakeholders involved in the decision, and what is the process in which those involved could come to a decision (e.g., what tools are/could be used to create an informed decision)?

   - Mark: What additional information do you think Mark needs?
   - Mark's parents: How can the advanced practice nurse support the parents?
   - Clinic: What are the policies for the clinic? Is the clinic affiliated with a mental health clinic? Does the health center have an ethics committee or access to a clinical ethicist?
   - Hospital PMHNP: What responsibility does she have for Mark's care?
   - Hospital SW who arranged discharge plan: What additional support can she provide the patient and family? Where else can she refer the patient?
   - State Board of Nursing (or APRN governance body in state): Is the care the FNP is providing within her scope of practice? What about for your state?
   - Local first responders (crisis team, law enforcement, EMS): Do first responders have the knowledge and skills to provide the appropriate care in your area to patients with mental health challenges?
   - Community members, neighbors: How can you educate your community about the mental health needs of patients like Mark?

4. What are the values relevant to this problem? *Values* are the things that you believe are important in making the decision. They (should) determine priorities. Values relevant to this problem may not be representative of your own personal values or moral framework.

   - The ethical principles of autonomy, beneficence, and non-maleficence often become incorporated into the values of providers. How are these three principles or values balanced against each other in this case?

   - Does accepting the LAI, even without fully informed consent and potentially coerced, help Mark achieve his goal of avoiding re-hospitalization?

   - Even if it does, do you have a right to violate his autonomy? Where is the line?

   - Does continuing these medications help maintain Mark's well-being in both the short term and long term, or does it potentially contribute to harm? Does it assist Mark's desire to avoid re-hospitalization?

   - Without medication, does Mark present a danger to himself or others? How so? Is the danger imminent?

5. What are the options for the decision? Think in terms of values and feasibility (e.g., financial, political, organizational, religious constraints).

   - Proceed as the APRN in this case study did?

   - Work to identify another psychiatric provider who can assume care?

   - Identify resources for psychiatric consultation to ensure that appropriate care is provided while bridging patient to community mental health center?

   - Stop prior to administering LAI and provide further education to Mark regarding the purpose of the injection including benefits, risks, and potential adverse effects?

   - Stop fluoxetine because it can contribute to mania and continue aripiprazole LAI only?

   - Decline to bridge the medications?

Management of Case Study

After all considerations, write a short narrative describing the best way to manage this situation; list core values important to you for managing the situation.

References

Appelbaum, P. S. (2007). Assessment of patients' competence to consent to treatment. *New England Journal of Medicine*, 357(18), 1834–1840. https://doi.org/10.1056/nejmcp074045

Balestra, M. L. (2019). Family nurse practitioner scope of practice issues when treating patients with mental health issues. *The Journal for Nurse Practitioners*, 15(7), 479–482. https://doi.org/10.1016/j.nurpra.2018.11.007

CASE STUDY #8

DEPRESSION SCREENING IN ADOLESCENTS

Depression in adolescents is a significant concern, as it can lead to negative health and social outcomes. Often, psychopharmacological solutions are immediately considered, as opposed to carefully considering environmental or interpersonal contributions to depression such as family dynamics, bullying, academic stressors, or social stressors and identifying how to help an adolescent better navigate and cope with these dynamics or challenges. By not considering these factors and addressing them, psychopharmacological intervention alone is unlikely to be effective.

Consider:

1. Identify the ethical concerns with this situation.

- Has Jake been accurately assessed and diagnosed?

- Is he receiving appropriate care?

- Laws are being enacted in some states that restrict practice regarding transgender care. If these laws exist in your state, how do they impact your ability to practice ethically?

- What is the ethical obligation of a provider if laws are enacted that interfere with evidence-based care? How does one navigate in these situations to care for their patients and also ensure that they maintain the ability to practice, do not violate laws, and ensure their own well-being?

- As a 14-year-old, is Jake entitled to autonomy as it pertains to medical decision-making? Age of consent for treatment varies by state. Do you know what your state's age of consent is?

- Are Jake's best interests being adequately addressed?

- Who decided Jake's best interest?

- Does lack of a policy absolve a provider from following practice guidelines, such as those published by the American Academy of Pediatrics?

- What is the ethical obligation of a provider if their practice setting is either not supportive of evidence-based guidelines or has policies and expectations inconsistent with evidence-based guidelines?

- The PHQ-A is a screening tool developed to screen for depression. It is not diagnostic, but it is being used as a diagnostic tool in this case to drive treatment. Other disorders or disease states may account for the elevated score on the PHQ-A and if not adequately ruled out may result in harm to Jake, as he could be receiving unnecessary treatment while the actual problems are not addressed. How should you use this screening tool, or should you use it at all?

2. What information will you need before a responsible decision can be made? (Consider what the information is and where it will come from.)

    - Is there a clinic policy or guideline regarding suicide assessment?

    - What supports are available in the clinic to Jake and his family to help support them in navigating his depression and needs around gender identity?

    - What are his actual height, weight, VS, orthostatic BP and HR, and labs assessing for electrolyte abnormalities, malnutrition, and endocrinopathies?

    - What resources are available regarding nutritional assessment or eating disorder assessment?

    - What resources are available at school for Jake?

    - Did Jake have an interest in pursuing counseling?

    - What are the insurance coverage and costs that need to be addressed for the father?

    - How are medical records of adolescents handled electronically with patient access? Do parents have immediate access to all the notes, or does it change during adolescence to block some information? Parents or legal guardians generally have the right to their child's health information (Dworkowitz, 2022). However, the immediate access to electronic records implemented as a response to the 21st Century Cures Act complicates this access for adolescents, as they do have a right to privacy and ability to consent to some services in some states (Dworkowitz, 2022). Access is often operationalized differently by different healthcare organizations. Do you know what your organization's or state's policy is? How can you find out?

3. Who are the stakeholders involved in the decision, and what is the process in which those involved could come to a decision (e.g., what tools are/could be used to create an informed decision)?

    - Jake: How can you best support the patient?

    - Jake's parents: How can you provide additional information to the parents and still maintain their trust?

- Clinic: Does the clinic have an ethics committee or access to a clinical ethicist? What resources and policies does the clinic need to support patients like Jake and his family?
- FNP: Is she providing care within her scope of practice? Does she have the information she needs to continue to provide care to Jake?

4. What are the values relevant to this problem? *Values* are the things that you believe are important in making the decision. They (should) determine priorities. Values relevant to this problem may not be representative of your own personal values or moral framework.

- Was adequate concern for Jake shown in this scenario?
- While the FNP treated Jake with respect during the visit, the lack of referral to appropriate services for support may result in being unable to access gender-affirming care in the future, which will ensure that even if he does not feel respected or valued by his parents, he will have increased potential to resources that will treat him with respect and compassion.
- The FNP treated Jake with compassion in the moment. However, what is the responsibility of the FNP to help ensure that he will continue to be treated in a compassionate manner?
- Would you consider the care that Jake received excellent? Why or why not?

5. What are the options for the decision? Think in terms of values and feasibility (e.g., financial, political, organizational, religious constraints).

- Should you complete a suicide risk assessment? While the PHQ-A demonstrated validity in screening for depressive symptoms, using a depression screening as a means to assess for suicide risk is inadequate (Horowitz et al., 2021).
- Should you complete a clinically appropriate assessment regarding Jake's significant weight loss (70% to 50% percentile)?
- When talking with Jake without his father present, in addition to asking about preferred pronouns, should you ask about treatment preferences such as counseling versus medication? What about ideas that he may have regarding maintaining confidentiality while he pursues treatment if he so desires?
- Should you offer referrals to local and online LGBTQIA resources when talking with Jake without his father present? Do your state laws and facility policies allow this?
- What laws does your state have regarding gender-affirming care?

Management of Case Study

After all considerations, write a short narrative describing the best way to manage this situation; list core values important to you for managing the situation.

References

Dworkowitz, A. (2022, May 16). Provider obligations for patient portals under the 21st Century Cures Act. *HealthAffairs*. https://doi.org/10.1377/forefront.20220513.923426

Horowitz, L. M., Mournet, A. M., Lanzillo, E., He, J.-P., Powell, D. S., Ross, A. M., Wharff, E. A., Bridge, J. A., & Pao, M. (2021). Screening pediatric medical patients for suicide risk: Is depression screening enough? *Journal of Adolescent Health*, *68*(6), 1183–1188. https://doi.org/10.1016/j.jadohealth.2021.01.028

CASE STUDY #9

TREATMENT OF RESISTANT ANXIETY

Carol experiences significant anxiety. She is also on a medication regimen that poses significant risks to her well-being and is inconsistent with treatment guidelines for the management of anxiety. Furthermore, her diagnosis of treatment resistant anxiety may not be accurate, as she may not have received effective treatment for anxiety in the past during the medication trials that appeared to have led to her anxiety being labeled "treatment resistant."

Consider:

1. Identify the ethical concerns with this situation.

    - What needs to be considered for Carol's medication in regards to potential harm, side effects, drug-drug interactions, and risks associated with her history of addiction?

    - Should Carol's medications be changed to a more evidence-based regimen to support their efficacy, which would likely improve her overall well-being?

    - Psycho-education as well as therapy are key factors in the treatment of anxiety (Anxiety & Depression Association of America, 2016). It is unclear if Carol has had significant opportunity to engage with psycho-education and therapy for treatment of her anxiety. Should you inquire about these interventions and make a referral?

2. What information will you need before a responsible decision can be made? (Consider what the information is and where it will come from.)

    - Can you confirm accuracy of past antidepressant trials for anxiety and Carol's response?

    - Is there a trusted provider who Carol may be more apt to receive information from with her current understanding of her diagnosis and treatment?

    - As Carol is involved in Narcotics Anonymous (NA), could her sponsor or a trusted person within NA be helpful in trying to motivate Carol to consider making a change?

3. Who are the stakeholders involved in the decision, and what is the process in which those involved could come to a decision (e.g., what tools are/could be used to create an informed decision)?

    - FNP: Does the FNP have the knowledge and skills to provide Carol's care?

    - Psychologist: What support and interventions can the psychologist provide to assist?

    - NA sponsor: Can you discuss the potential of Carol's NA sponsor supporting her in making medication changes?

    - Health insurance: Some companies disincentivize prescribing practices such as Carol's regimen. How can you assure Carol will be able to receive her medications?

4. What are the values relevant to this problem? *Values* are the things that you believe are important in making the decision. They (should) determine priorities. Values relevant to this problem may not be representative of your own personal values or moral framework.

    - Safety: Carol's medication regimen presents a variety of risks to her health and well-being. How can you provide a safer regimen?

    - Commitment to excellence in care: The PMHNP demonstrates a commitment to excellence as demonstrated by the conversation she had with Carol regarding the risks of her medications and recommendations. However, if Carol is not willing to make changes in the future, what is the PMHNP's responsibility?

5. What are the options for the decision? Think in terms of values and feasibility (e.g., financial, political, organizational, religious constraints).

    - Continue prescribing the current medication regimen to avoid angering Carol, as it has been working thus far?

    - See how Carol does with engaging in therapy and if it is effective?

    - Begin to taper clonazepam and tell Carol that if she is not in agreement, she can find a new psychiatric provider?

    - Offer more education regarding duloxetine and average BP increase?

Management of Case Study

After all considerations, write a short narrative describing the best way to manage this situation; list core values important to you for managing the situation.

Reference

Anxiety & Depression Association of America. (2016, March 16). *Clinical practice review for GAD.* https://adaa.org/resources-professionals/practice-guidelines-gad

CASE STUDY #10

COVID-19 VACCINE IN ADOLESCENCE

The CDC recommends the COVID vaccine for 12- to 15-year-olds, and significant data have indicated that it is safe and effective for this group. But in most states, parental consent is required for children and adolescents less than 18 years old to receive vaccinations. What should you do when a 15-year-old seeks vaccination but does not want his parents to know?

Consider:

1. Identify the ethical concerns with this situation.

    - Does the FNP educate Barry about the vaccine but not provide the vaccine since his parents are not there to provide consent?

    - Does the FNP call and discuss Barry's request with the parents?

    - Does the FNP provide the family with education concerning the vaccine?

    - Who else is at risk if the vaccine is not provided?

    - How can you maintain Barry's trust and still follow the legal requirements of the state?

2. What information will you need before a responsible decision can be made? (Consider what the information is and where it will come from.)

    - What is the health literacy of the parents? Where do they receive their information regarding vaccines?

    - Where are the CDC guidelines for you to access? Can you provide this information to Barry and his parents?

    - Would information from the friend's father assist in the discussion?

- What is the advanced practice nurse's role in the discussion? Is it to persuade the parents or inform?

3. Who are the stakeholders involved in the decision, and what is the process in which those involved could come to a decision (e.g., what tools are/could be used to create an informed decision)?

    - Patient: How can you alleviate his fear about getting COVID if you are unable to vaccinate him?
    - Parents: What information do you need to educate his parents about COVID and the vaccine?
    - Advanced practice nurse : What additional knowledge does the FNP need? Are there tools the advanced practice nurse could use to help with the conversation about the vaccine? What are they?
        - Centers for Disease Control and Prevention
        - Vaccine information statement
        - Motivational interviewing
        - World Health Organization
        - Shared decision-making tools

4. What are the values relevant to this problem? *Values* are the things that you believe are important in making the decision. They (should) determine priorities. Values relevant to this problem may not be representative of your own personal values or moral framework.

    - How can you support Barry and also abide by the policies and law in California?
    - How can the advanced practice nurse establish trust with Barry and his parents?
    - What guidance does Barry need to protect his autonomy?

5. What are the options for the decision? Think in terms of values and feasibility (e.g., financial, political, organizational, religious constraints).

    - Do Barry and his parents have the health literacy and information required about the vaccine?
    - Are there any religious considerations?
    - Are there any financial considerations?
    - Are there any requirements of the organization that would prevent the advanced practice nurse from engaging the parents?

Management of Case Study

After all considerations, write a short narrative describing the best way to manage this situation; list core values important to you for managing the situation.

CASE STUDY #11

MEDICAL EMANCIPATION VERSUS CONFIDENTIALITY IN TRANSGENDER AND GENDER-NONCONFORMING PEOPLE

This case study represents the complexity of caring for transgender and gender-nonconforming people, especially those who are adolescents with parents unaware of their struggles.

Consider:

1. Identify the ethical concerns with this situation.

    - How do you protect Luna's autonomy and respect his confidentiality?

    - How do you provide care and respect Luna's parents and their religious beliefs?

    - Laws are being enacted in some states that restrict practice regarding transgender care. If these laws exist in your state, how do they impact your ability to practice ethically?

    - What is the ethical obligation of a provider if laws are enacted that interfere with evidence-based care? How does one navigate in these situations to care for their patients and also ensure that they maintain the ability to practice, do not violate laws, and ensure their own well-being?

    - What healthcare organizational policies exist for this type of situation? Do they conflict with evidence-based guidelines?

2. What information will you need before a responsible decision can be made? (Consider what the information is and where it will come from.)

- What are the practice guidelines from the American Academy of Pediatrics, and where can you find them?

- Is there a clinic policy or guidelines regarding the care of transgender and gender non-conforming children? Does a lack of a policy absolve a provider from following practice guidelines, such as those published by the American Academy of Pediatrics?

- What support does the clinic offer for the patient and the family regarding gender identity?

- Are resources available at the school for Luna?

- Is counseling available for Luna and his parents?

- Does the health insurance provide coverage/cost for counseling?

- What is the state law regarding restriction or non-restriction of practice concerning transgender and gender non-conforming youth?

- How are medical records of adolescents handled? Do adolescents have a right to privacy and ability to consent in Luna's state? How will this complicate his care?

3. Who are the stakeholders involved in the decision, and what is the process in which those involved could come to a decision (e.g., what tools are/could be used to create an informed decision)?

- Patient: How do you support him and provide the care he needs?

- Parents: What information does Louisa need for today's visit?

- Advanced practice nurse: What information does the FNP need to continue to provide care to Luna?

- Clinic/healthcare organization: What policies does the clinic have regarding transgender youth? Are there laws in Idaho that might hinder the care Luna needs?

4. What are the values relevant to this problem? *Values* are the things that you believe are important in making the decision. They (should) determine priorities. Values relevant to this problem may not be representative of your own personal values or moral framework.

- How do you advocate for Luna?

- Can the advanced practice nurse establish trust with Luna? With his parents?

- How do you provide a safe environment for Luna?

5. What are the options for the decision? Think in terms of values and feasibility (e.g., financial, political, organizational, religious constraints).

- Do Luna and his parents have the health literacy and information required about transgender and gender non-conforming people to make decisions?

- Are there any religious considerations?

- Are there any financial considerations?

- Are there any requirements of the state or the healthcare organization that would prevent the advanced practice nurse from advocating for Luna?

Management of Case Study

After all considerations, write a short narrative describing the best way to manage this situation; list core values important to you for managing the situation.

CASE STUDY #12

CHILDHOOD OBESITY

This case study addresses the increasing health concern of childhood obesity and its long-term consequences to children.

Consider:

1. Identify the ethical concerns with this situation.

    - Is the provider struggling with who is responsible?

    - How do you address this health issue with the mother in the time allotted? Do you sign off on the permission slip for baseball without addressing the child's obesity?

2. What information will you need before a responsible decision can be made? (Consider what the information is and where it will come from.)

    - What actions have been taken previously by the provider and the family?

    - What information is available about the school Isaac attends and the community where he lives?

    - What about the availability of grocery stores, fresh fruit and vegetables, farmer's markets, accessible meal preparation classes, and transportation?

    - What other influences are there on Isaac: friends and relatives?

3. Who are the stakeholders involved in the decision, and what is the process in which those involved could come to a decision (e.g., what tools are/could be used to create an informed decision)?

    - How should the FNP think about this situation?

    - Isaac: Do you need to engage Isaac?

- Provider: What guidelines are most appropriate for this situation? Where do you find them?

- Gloria: Have the growth charts been shown to Isaac's mother Gloria?

- Provider: Where would the provider find evidence-based data to support the facts on obesity as "socially contagious"? How would you incorporate this data into the conversation?

- Parents: Does the father need to be involved?

- Clinic/healthcare organization: What about the clinic? Or other providers?

4. What are the values relevant to this problem? *Values* are the things that you believe are important in making the decision. They (should) determine priorities. Values relevant to this problem may not be representative of your own personal values or moral framework.

    - Does the provider need to have humility and compassion in this situation?

    - Is the provider's responsibility to be honest with Gloria and Isaac about his weight and the lifelong impact obesity will have on his health?

    - What are the best ways to connect with the family to have the best chance of making an impact?

5. What are the options for the decision? Think in terms of values and feasibility (e.g., financial, political, organizational, religious constraints).

    - What opportunities exist in the community or at the clinic that can assist Gloria and the family?

    - Again, knowing that obesity is "socially contagious," how can you use this information to assist you moving forward with a plan of care for this family?

Management of Case Study

After all considerations, write a short narrative describing the best way to manage this situation; list core values important to you for managing the situation.

CASE STUDY #13

DEMENTIA AND STOPPING DRIVING

When Janet was hospitalized, she experienced delirium, which is also sometimes called an acute confusional state. Due to the delirium, she experienced confusion and changes in behavior that appeared to have led to concerns regarding her cognitive functioning, as a MoCA was done during her admission. Additionally, a doctor made a recommendation that she does not drive, which her son took seriously by removing her car keys. The FNP is now in the position of trying to determine if it is safe for Janet to be driving.

Consider:

1. What are the ethical concerns with this situation? List them and the elements that should be considered in this case study.

    - Maintaining the privilege to drive is an instrumental part of helping many older individuals maintain their sense of autonomy. What are the elements of autonomy to be considered in this case study?

    - Removing Janet's driving privileges may result in increasing her safety and the safety of her community and thus ensuring that harm is not done to others. However, it may also result in unnecessary harm by unnecessarily limiting her independence and freedom if Janet is indeed safe to drive. What are the elements of non-maleficence to be considered in this case study?

    - Helping Janet maintain her driving privileges, if she is safe to do so, can actually help maintain her health and well-being by making it easier for her to continue to be an active member of her community and to engage with her healthcare providers. What are the elements of beneficence to be considered in this case study?

2. What information will you need before a responsible decision can be made? (Consider what the information is and where it will come from.)

- What additional information do you need about Janet's functional abilities?
- Does her vision or hearing impair her ability to drive?
- Does she have any mobility issues that would impair her ability to drive?
- What information regarding her ability to react to unforeseen circumstances while driving do you need to consider?
- Distractibility and deficits in attention are a hallmark of delirium, and individuals do not always return to their previous baseline functioning. Does this apply to Janet?
- Cognitive testing does not necessarily correlate with functional abilities; therefore, updated cognitive testing may be nice, but is it necessary?
- Was a mandatory report made to the DMV by a previous provider?
- Are there resources available to you to help with this decision such as an occupational therapist (OT) or programs for senior drivers through the DMV or auto insurance?
- Does her son have any concerns other than what was mentioned briefly during her admission regarding driving?
- Did Janet get anything in the mail from the DMV indicating a report was made regarding concern about her ability to continue driving?
- Prior to her hospitalization, had Janet begun to curtail her driving on her own due to discomfort or perceived limitations, such as avoiding rush hour, abstaining from driving at night, or not driving to unfamiliar locations?

3. Who are the stakeholders involved in the decision, and what is the process in which those involved could come to a decision (e.g., what tools are/could be used to create an informed decision)?

- Janet: What does Janet think about this decision? Have you included them in the discussion?
- Janet's son: What does Janet's son think about this decision? Have you included them in the discussion?
- Doctor who made recommendation to son regarding not driving: What are the provider's responsibilities in this situation? What is the provider's role?
- OT: What are the OT's responsibilities in this situation?
- DMV: What tools does the DMV need to determine the outcome in this situation? What is the role of the DMV?
- Auto insurance company: What is covered by auto insurance regarding this situation?

4. What are the values relevant to this problem? *Values* are the things that you believe are important in making the decision. They (should) determine priorities. Values relevant to this problem may not be representative of your own personal values or moral framework.

- Safety for Janet and her community: What considerations must be considered?

- Independence: Driving helps Janet maintain her independence. What are ways for Janet to maintain her independence after this decision?

- Freedom: Driving helps Janet maintain a level of freedom she may not feel otherwise. What are ways for Janet to maintain her freedom after this decision?

- Fun: Driving helps Janet continue the activities she finds enjoyable. What other ways does Janet have fun?

- Community: Driving helps Janet maintain a sense of community and decreases isolation. How will Janet maintain community moving forward?

- Balance: If it is unsafe for Janet to drive, how will the above-mentioned values be maintained? Are they as important as safety?

- Excellence in practice: What is the most evidence-based methodology for going about removing someone's driving privileges in this scenario?

5. What are the options for the decision? Think in terms of values and feasibility (e.g., financial, political, organizational, religious constraints).

- Recommend that Janet continue not to drive because the doctor in the hospital said, "It probably isn't safe for Janet to drive anymore"?

- Recommend that Janet resume driving because the conditions that led to the doctor recommending that "it probably isn't safe for Janet to drive anymore" appear to be resolved?

- Refer to the OT for additional assessment regarding Janet's functional abilities?

- Recommend that Janet spend some time driving with her son to see if he has any concerns about her ability to drive?

- Recommend that Janet continue to refrain from driving while you attempt to ascertain if a report was indeed made to the DMV?

- Learn more about Janet's driving to see if a plan can be made to allow some driving but minimizing more dangerous aspects of driving or aspects that she may find challenging, such as only driving during the day or only driving to familiar locations?

Management of Case Study

After all considerations, write a short narrative describing the best way to manage this situation; list core values important to you for managing the situation.

CASE STUDY #14

WHEN TO TRANSITION TO PALLIATIVE CARE

This case study highlights the complexity of medical decision-making in the context of serious illness. Communication with patients and families is an ongoing process that may involve ethical dilemmas.

Consider:

1. Identify the ethical concerns with this situation.

    - If the goal is to "do no harm," what is considered the least harmful choice?

    - How does one weigh the risks and benefits of each treatment option?

    - Who should the decision-maker in this case be?

2. What information will you need before a responsible decision can be made? (Consider what the information is and where it will come from.)

    - What are the state laws regarding surrogate decision-making?

    - Does Katie's cousin have any insights about her wishes that she may have shared with him in conversation?

3. Who are the stakeholders involved in the decision, and what is the process in which those involved could come to a decision (e.g., what tools are/could be used to create an informed decision)?

    - Katie: What are Katie's thoughts? What does she think about this situation?

    - Katie's parents: What do they think about this situation?

- Katie's cousin: What does Katie's cousin think?

- Are there cultural and/or religious considerations?

- Medical providers: Can communication tools be used to assess family understanding of the situation during the family meeting? Ideally, a family meeting should include a pre-briefing and de-briefing among providers.

- What questions for each stakeholder should be considered?

4. What are the values relevant to this problem? *Values* are the things that you believe are important in making the decision. They (should) determine priorities. Values relevant to this problem may not be representative of your own personal values or moral framework.

    - What healthcare resources are being utilized to provide care to Katie?

    - What potential harm could come to Katie depending on healthcare decisions that are made?

    - What are Katie's values related to healthcare decision-making?

    - How are her family members' and healthcare providers' positions informed by their own values?

    - Consider autonomy, distributive justice, beneficence, and non-maleficence.

    - What questions for each value should be considered?

5. What are the options for the decision? Think in terms of values and feasibility (e.g., financial, political, organizational, religious constraints).

    - Who should be at the table for the family meeting?

    - Should an ethics committee be consulted?

    - Should legal be consulted?

    - Should we proceed with resection? Should we shift to comfort measures only?

Management of Case Study

After all considerations, write a short narrative describing the best way to manage this situation; list core values important to you for managing the situation.

CASE STUDY #15

PRESCRIPTION REFILL DILEMMA FOR PATIENT AND SPOUSE IN FINANCIAL STRAITS

This case study represents the all-too-familiar occurrence of patients with and without health insurance trying to manage their care with the overwhelming burden of the cost of their medications. In this couple with limited income and similar medical problems, one has insurance and the other does not.

Consider:

1. Identify the ethical concerns with this situation.
    - Who would be harmed in this situation?
    - How do you empathize with Tony but protect your license?
    - What does the state law in your state require regarding prescribing to family members?
    - Do you ignore Tony's request while being aware that his wife is unable to manage her disease due to financial concerns?

2. What information will you need before a responsible decision can be made? (Consider what the information is and where it will come from.)
    - What are the treatment guidelines for diabetes care? Do you have access to them and know where to find them?
    - Do you also manage Marline's care? Might a joint appointment benefit both of them? Would reconciling the medications of both assist with the decision?
    - What policies are in place in the clinic that could assist you?
    - Is a patient assistance program available for both?

- Does the clinic have a social worker that could assist with the financial management needed for the medications?

3. Who are the stakeholders involved in the decision, and what is the process in which those involved could come to a decision (e.g., what tools are/could be used to create an informed decision)?

    - Tony: What does Tony think about this situation?
    - Marline: What does Tony's wife think about this situation?
    - Nurse practitioner: What is the role of the NP? What elements does the NP need to consider? What is the scope of practice for the NP in this situation? What about in your state?
    - Clinic: What is the clinic's role? What about liability? Health of patient?
    - Community: Are there additional clinical resources in the community such as a free clinic that offers medications?

4. What are the values relevant to this problem? *Values* are the things that you believe are important in making the decision. They (should) determine priorities. Values relevant to this problem may not be representative of your own personal values or moral framework.

    - Does the provider need to have humility and compassion in this situation?
    - Is the provider's responsibility to be honest with Tony and Marline regarding the legal constraints that the nurse practitioner faces?
    - What is the best way to connect with the couple to have the best chance of making an impact?

5. What are the options for the decision? Think in terms of values and feasibility (e.g., financial, political, organizational, religious constraints).

    - Reconcile the medications for both to see where medications overlap or are redundant? Are older, less-costly medications an option? What are the American Diabetes Association diabetes guidelines? Do they offer solutions you hadn't thought of?
    - Refer both to a patient assistance program?
    - Refer both to community clinics that offer assistance for medications or to GoodRx?
    - Maximize benefits offered by the clinic?
    - Who can provide social justice and advocacy for patients like Tony and Marline?

Management of Case Study

After all considerations, write a short narrative describing the best way to manage this situation; list core values important to you for managing the situation.

CASE STUDY #16

CRNA LABOR AND DELIVERY EPIDURAL PAIN MANAGEMENT WITH A LANGUAGE BARRIER

This case study presents several issues that concern the safe administration of anesthesia to women during childbirth.

Consider:

1. Identify the ethical concerns with this situation.

    - Can you provide anesthesia care in the hallway?

    - Who is responsible for monitoring the patient?

    - What about the language barrier?

    - What about the lack of prenatal care? Is the labor & delivery (L&D) staff prepared for deliveries outside of the labor room setting (hallway, lounge, parking lot)?

    - Where does the nexus of ethical concerns intersect for the L&D nurse, the physician on duty, and the CRNA? What happens if this patient experiences a precipitous delivery, prolonged labor, fetal distress, or postpartum bleeding?

    - How do you reconcile patient safety, patient comfort, and patient privacy issues?

2. What information will you need before a responsible decision can be made? (Consider what the information is and where it will come from.)

    - What are the guidelines to follow?

- What are your professional and organizational resources for decision-making?
- Is there additional information you need from Dolores? What about her cousin?
- What information can the L&D nurses provide?
- What information can the ED physician and/or the OB physician (or the OB attending) provide to assist in decision-making?
- Can the Nurse Supervisor give clarity on unit staffing issues and L&D room availability?

3. Who are the stakeholders involved in the decision, and what is the process in which those involved could come to a decision (e.g., what tools are/could be used to create an informed decision)?
   - Patient: What does the patient think in this situation? Have you included them in the discussion?
   - CRNA: What is the scope and role of the CRNA?
   - Healthcare organization: What is the role of the healthcare organization?
   - Licensing boards: What is the role of the state licensing board?
   - Besides the patient and the CRNA, who are additional stakeholders?

4. What are the values relevant to this problem? *Values* are the things that you believe are important in making the decision. They (should) determine priorities. Values relevant to this problem may not be representative of your own personal values or moral framework.
   - Does the provider need to have humility and compassion in this situation?
   - Is the provider's responsibility to be honest with Dolores?
   - How do you inform the patient of her situation and choices in a culturally respectful and knowledgeable way?
   - How does the language barrier impact your ability to obtain informed consent and ensure that the patient understands her situation?
   - How do you best respect the patient's privacy in a hallway?
   - How do you establish a trusting relationship with the patient?

5. What are the options for the decision? Think in terms of values and feasibility (e.g., financial, political, organizational, religious constraints).
   - Are there protocols in place in the childbirth center that prevent the use of hallways for anesthesia procedures?
   - What can you do to prevent future occurrences?
   - What opportunities exist in the community or at the clinic that can assist Dolores and her family?

Management of Case Study

After all considerations, write a short narrative describing the best way to manage this situation; list core values important to you for managing the situation.

CASE STUDY #17

VIOLENCE, SUICIDE, AND FAMILY DYNAMICS WITH MEDICAL COMPLEXITY

Peter was initially determined to be at imminent risk for suicide and placed on a "hold" to detain him in the hospital for observation due to concerns for his safety related to mental illness. However, Peter has significant medical comorbidities that have the potential to contribute to behavioral changes unrelated to potential mental illness. Additionally, during his hospitalization, Peter's mental status cleared without significant treatment, leading to concern that the events leading up to his admission may not have been consistent with those presented by his family. Lastly, Peter voiced concern that his family was trying to ensure that he remains in the hospital so they could take his money and property.

Consider:

1. Identify the ethical concerns with this situation.

   - In this case, no matter what clinical decision you make, is there a potential likelihood of harm to Peter or a member of his family?

   - How do you provide a benefit in this case? What type of benefit—clinical benefit, community benefit, psychological/emotional benefit? For whom are you responsible for providing a benefit: Is it Peter, his family, the community, the hospital?

   - Is Peter his own decision-maker and does he have a right to engage in making decisions regarding his care, living arrangements, and goals?

- What represents justice in this case? Is it Peter getting to live the last few months of his life consistent with how he would want and dying how he would want? Or is it ensuring that others feel safe from him? Is Peter not able to obtain home health services such as hospice because his medical record now describes him as "violent" and "suicidal" with potential access to firearms, even though the claims were not substantiated and he made suicidal statements, but his only action was to walk into the garage?

2. What information will you need before a responsible decision can be made? (Consider what the information is and where it will come from.)

    - In many if not most cases, it is impossible to obtain all the information you would like before coming to a responsible decision. In this case, that is especially true, as you are receiving conflicting information from different parties without having the ability to verify the information. Both Peter and his family may be motivated to be dishonest. As much as providers may like to believe they are skilled at determining who is being truthful and who is not, this is typically not an accurate assumption. How can you get all the information you need to make a decision while keeping these realities in mind?
    - Did Peter really start fires in the home with his wife's belongings on the floor?
    - Was Peter abusive to his wife and family as described by his daughter?
    - Has Peter made any verifiable threats to anyone or himself?
    - Has Peter ever made any other suicidal statements or had any past history of suicidal behavior?
    - How independent was Peter prior to admission? The information provided by his daughter seemed to change over time and is inconsistent with how Peter described himself.
    - Are Peter's cognitive and behavioral changes related to his medical comorbidities, medication side effects, stress, a psychiatric diagnosis, or a combination thereof? Is it even possible to know?
    - Does he have a past history of depression, anxiety, or PTSD?
    - Does Peter have decisional capacity?
    - Are there other family members or friends who Peter would want involved in his care?
    - What are Peter's goals and wishes?
    - How has Peter navigated significant challenges in his life in the past?
    - Does Peter actually have access to firearms outside the hospital?
    - If Peter is discharged home, how would he be supported if his family is no longer there? Does he need caregiver support?
    - If Peter is discharged home with minimal support, how will he get to his ongoing outpatient medical appointments? Is he capable of driving? Does he have access to medical transportation?

3. Who are the stakeholders involved in the decision, and what is the process in which those involved could come to a decision (e.g., what tools are/could be used to create an informed decision)?

   - Peter: What does Peter think happened? Who does Peter think is responsible?

   - Primary team (intern, resident, attending): What is the role of the primary team?

   - Peter's oncologist: What is the role of Peter's oncologist?

   - County pre-commitment investigative team: Can they help verify some information and collaborate regarding need for ongoing hospitalization and treatment?

   - Peter's daughter and son-in-law and potentially other family members whom he could identify to be involved in his care: Who are the important family members? What is their role in care?

   - Adult Protective Services: There appears to be grounds for mandatory reporting due to Peter's claim that family is trying to ensure that he remains in the hospital to take his money and property. Also of concern is his statement regarding his daughter feeding him one meal a day and his questioning if she was doing something with his medications. These accusations about food deprivation and medication tampering could potentially be corroborated by his clinical improvement while hospitalized with minimal intervention other than regular food and fluids and being restarted on his home medications. Should Adult Protective Services be brought into this case?

   - Social work: Can they provide assistance with disposition planning, safety planning, and other resources?

   - Care management: Can they provide assistance with home services and hospice information should Peter desire it?

   - Palliative care: What elements does palliative care need to consider?

   - Law enforcement: Is there a duty to warn requiring notification to law enforcement? Or, since law enforcement responded to the home and brought the patient in, could they help provide collateral information? In some jurisdictions, elder abuse reports may also be made directly to law enforcement rather than to Adult Protective Services, depending on the nature of the complaint or the time of day.

   - Hospital risk management: Should you review the case with risk management? In cases as complicated as this, risk management can often be helpful to ensure that you are not missing anything.

   - Clinical ethics: Is there an ethics service available? Reviewing a complex case such as this with an ethics service is often helpful to clarify ethical responsibilities of providers and caregivers.

4. What are the values relevant to this problem? *Values* are the things that you believe are important in making the decision. They (should) determine priorities. Values relevant to this problem may not be representative of your own personal values or moral framework.

   - How can you balance Peter's safety and the safety of his family, the community, and hospital employees?

- For whatever reason, it appears that not all the involved parties in this case were being completing truthful. As a provider you have no means to force people to tell the truth, but you have an obligation to make the best decisions you can with the information you have and attempt to find the truth within the information provided. How do you manage this?

- Peter is dying and has little time left to live. How is it possible to help him be comfortable (physically and emotionally) during his last few months while also ensuring that he and others are safe? This may seem extraneous, but ensuring this will likely help mitigate the risk of violence toward self and others.

- What does it mean for Peter to have a meaningful last few months of life and a meaningful death? Is this something he is interested in exploring?

- Prior to assuming one's symptoms are related to a psychiatric disorder, medical causes of symptoms must be considered and ruled out if possible. This appeared to have been done in this case, with a workup for paraneoplastic encephalitis being considered and determined low-yield due to inability to surgically remove or treat cancer, as well as provide improvement in the patient's symptoms. What are other factors that need to be considered in this case for the PMHNP? Did the PMHNP prescribe medications without clear benefit?

- Patient initially consented to involve his daughter in his care. Should this be revisited? What obligation does the team have to continue to communicate with the daughter? What obligation or right does the team have to communicate with others regarding the patient's care and condition—i.e., law enforcement, home health providers, etc? Should the team have stopped communication with the daughter when her communication appeared to inflame matters?

5. What are the options for the decision? Think in terms of values and feasibility (e.g., financial, political, organizational, religious constraints).

- Refrain from recommending discharge as recommended by primary team and family due to their voiced safety concerns despite lack of legal grounds to detain patient and his right to discharge? This is not a recommended option but would alleviate the discomfort of the primary team temporarily and potentially result in fewer complaints from the family. It is, however, a violation of the patient's civil rights.

- Prescribe antipsychotic for irritability and antidepressant for management of PTSD as asked to by primary team to alleviate concerns of providers and staff? Again, this is not a recommended option; however, antipsychotics are frequently used for the management of behavioral disturbance in individuals with cognitive impairment, though their use is off label, and there are significant risks associated with their use (Meeks & Jeste, 2008). Additionally, while antidepressants are often viewed as benign medications, there does not seem to be an indication that Peter is experiencing a major depressive episode. He is more likely experiencing a psychological response to illness, which an antidepressant would be unlikely to mediate. Furthermore, Peter seemed to have an adverse reaction to duloxetine in that he described it making him "nuttier than a bedbug." Lastly, an SSRI would take 6–8 weeks to reach full effect after being titrated to a therapeutic dose. While Peter may live longer than the three months predicted, he is unlikely to receive much benefit from an SSRI, and they do have side effects such as headache, GI upset, increased risk of bleeding, and hyponatremia.

- Admit Peter to inpatient psychiatry before the "hold" expires as pressured to do by primary team and family and let the inpatient psychiatry staff sort out the disposition problems and conflicting information? While this option would alleviate provider and family distress, it would not actually solve any problems. It is passing the challenge to a different team that is not familiar with the patient. Peter would need to be discharged when his "hold" expired. He does not appear to have an acute psychiatric disorder requiring inpatient psychiatric treatment; rather, he is experiencing significant stressors related to a terminal illness, family discord, and separation from his wife. None of this would be mediated by inpatient psych or psychopharmacological intervention. Counseling may help Peter modify his coping strategies, come to terms with his impending death, and modify his behavior; however, he would be better served in an outpatient setting where he could develop a relationship with someone who would work with him over time, not over a couple of days in an acute care setting.

- Make a report to Adult Protective Services regarding concerns for possible financial exploitation? Peter said his family is trying to ensure that he remains in the hospital so they can take his money and his property, and their behavior does seem somewhat consistent with the daughter's story. Additionally, it was reported that Peter stated he was being given one meal a day, and he was concerned that his daughter was doing something with his medications, as he feels so much better now despite supposedly being on the same medications.

- Complete a capacity evaluation to determine Peter's decisional capacity?

- Work with Peter to identify what family members or friends he would like to involve in his care and discharge planning and then work with them to gather additional collateral information and create a safe enough discharge plan?

- If Peter is determined to have capacity, only communicate with those he gives consent for you to do so?

- Ensure that a safety plan is completed regarding suicidal behaviors?

- Prior to discharge, complete duty to warn as allowed or required in your state? As access to firearms and veracity of threats prior to admission were never clarified, grounds for duty to warn do exist for notification to both family and local law enforcement. To family, provide date and times of discharge, and to law enforcement, provide minimally necessary information for them to be able to determine next steps for an investigation? This is typically patient's name, DOB, address, nature of safety concern warranting duty to warn, and date and time of discharge. You can also describe steps you have taken to help mitigate safety risk such as attempt to verify access to firearms and safety planning. If choosing this option, have you completed appropriate documentation as required by your organization when completing duty to warn and mandated reporting?

- Ensure that Peter is provided with referrals to outpatient services as consistent with his needs, goals, and values (e.g., counseling, hospice, home health)?

Management of Case Study

After all considerations, write a short narrative describing the best way to manage this situation; list core values important to you for managing the situation.

Reference

Meeks, T. W., & Jeste, D. V. (2008). Beyond the black box: What is the role for antipsychotics in dementia? *Current Psychiatry*, 7(6), 50–65.

CASE STUDY #18

PSYCHIATRIC ACUTE CONCERNS AND FALL RISKS

Marilyn is an 82-year-old woman with multiple falls at home prior to admission, who recently moved into assisted living and is having increased agitation resulting in the staff calling 911 and having her transported to the emergency department (ED). ED social work did not feel psychiatric admission was warranted. Marilyn was admitted to a medical ward, as her facility was not willing to take her back initially. In the hospital she became increasingly agitated, resulting in administration of IM antipsychotics, mechanical restraints, and eventually placement in a net enclosure bed due to her risk of falls to help ensure her safety.

Consider:

1. Identify the ethical concerns with this situation.

   - In preventing potential harm from potential falls through the use of bed alarms, keeping Marilyn in bed, and eventually the net-enclosure bed, are we causing more harm through isolation, deconditioning, and not allowing Marilyn to be as active as she is capable of?

   - What good do we provide Marilyn if while not falling, she becomes so deconditioned she can no longer walk or so isolated she becomes further disoriented?

   - Assisted living facilities have a responsibility to provide safe environments to their residents, but do they have the right to say they will not take their residents back unless conditions are met that are not deemed medically necessary by the treating providers at the hospital, such as inpatient psychiatric admission and assessment by geriatric psychiatry?

2. What information will you need before a responsible decision can be made? (Consider what the information is and where it will come from.)

    - What evidence-based interventions are available to minimize falls and risk of injury to patients with history of multiple falls prior to admission while helping them maintain their previous level of functioning and independence?

    - What are the criteria for the use of net-enclosure beds at this hospital?

    - What was Marilyn's baseline prior to admission and prior to her fall when she hit her head?

    - What has her course of improvement been like after hitting her head?

    - What are individualized measures that can be used with Marilyn to help prevent agitation—non-pharmacological interventions unique to her such as favorite music and other likes and dislikes?

    - What other resources are available within the hospital to help prevent Marilyn from falling, to de-escalate any agitated behaviors, and to help improve her strength?

3. Who are the stakeholders involved in the decision, and what is the process in which those involved could come to a decision (e.g., what tools are/could be used to create an informed decision)?

    - Marilyn: What are Marilyn's thoughts? Have they been included in the discussion?

    - Marilyn's daughter: What are Marilyn's daughter's thoughts? Have they been included in the discussion?

    - Nursing administrators: Beyond nursing unit leadership, what other nursing administrators need to be involved?

    - Nursing education: Is the net-enclosure bed being used appropriately? Are there other tools that can be implemented to help prevent falls in this case?

    - Primary team and cross-cover teams: Can they attempt to put in place a plan to prevent extraneous ordering of net-enclosure beds?

    - Pharmacy: There is a lot of pressure to "fix" Marilyn's behaviors with medication adjustments. Should pharmacy be brought in to assist with medication review and supporting PMHNP in the desire to limit medications rather than contribute to polypharmacy?

    - Clinical ethics: Would an ethics consultation be helpful in discerning the choices providers have and the risks associated with each choice to help choose a clinical path forward? For example, it may be ethically justifiable to allow for increased freedom of movement, mobility, and independence to maintain independence and functioning, even if that choice is associated with a risk of falling and injury if it is consistent with a patient's goals and values. However, while this may be the ethically justifiable approach, it may not be consistent with the goals of the hospital in terms of meeting quality metrics and reimbursement, and therefore may not be feasible.

4. What are the values relevant to this problem? *Values* are the things that you believe are important in making the decision. They (should) determine priorities. Values relevant to this problem may not be representative of your own personal values or moral framework.

- How can the provider balance Marilyn's safety (from falls and also from delirium) and the safety of staff?

- What are the guidelines for hospital reimbursement for care associated with an injury from a fall?

- A one-to-one may help Marilyn not fall, though there is no evidence that they prevent falls. However, use of one-to-ones stresses the healthcare system further and is a financial burden. Is such a use of resources appropriate in this case?

- How can you help Marilyn maintain as much independence as possible and her prior level of functioning while still considering other factors such as safety, excellence in care, and respect?

- How can you provide care in a manner consistent with available evidence and best practices?

- How can you care for Marilyn in a manner that demonstrates respect?

5. What are the options for the decision? Think in terms of values and feasibility (e.g., financial, political, organizational, religious constraints).

- Adjust medications as PMHNP and FNP did in this case?

- Decline to defer to geriatric psychiatry?

- Decline to prescribe medications as requested by ALF (lotion prepared by compounding pharmacy)?

- Order PT for frequent engagement with Marilyn, and reach out to clearly communicate goals of PT to ensure that order is not dismissed due to lack of clear understanding of Marilyn's functional baseline?

- Order OT for cognitive enrichment activities?

- Work with nursing leadership on unit to create a plan to get Marilyn out of net-enclosure bed with increased opportunities for restorative nursing activities and cognitive enrichment?

- Refer to inpatient psychiatry as requested by ALF and primary team, and let the inpatient psychiatry unit stabilize Marilyn's delirium? This is an option, though not recommended, as the underlying cause of Marilyn's behavior does not appear to be psychiatric in nature from information available, and it is not clear that inpatient psychiatry would be of any benefit to her.

Management of Case Study

After all considerations, write a short narrative describing the best way to manage this situation; list core values important to you for managing the situation.

CASE STUDY #19

TELEHEALTH

Case A: Urgent Referrals in Telehealth

This case addresses some of the ethical concerns faced by providers delivering care virtually. The desire of the provider and the patient often do not align. The provider is encouraged to think through how to manage this "misalignment" when not in physical space with the patient.

Consider:

1. Identify the ethical concerns with this situation.

    - What is the biggest concern for the patient? What are the relevant facts, laws, and principles?

    - What is the biggest concern for the provider? What are the relevant facts, laws, and principles?

2. What information will you need before a responsible decision can be made? (Consider what the information is and where it will come from.)

    - Are there any clinic policies or procedures in place that would help you address this issue/concern?

    - Could there be facts in this case that you are unaware of?

3. Who are the stakeholders involved in the decision, and what is the process in which those involved could come to a decision (e.g., what tools are/could be used to create an informed decision)?

    - Consumer groups: Are there consumer groups that might have input into this particular issue? What about family or friends?

    - Resources: Are there other resources you could offer the patient?

    - Additional assistance: Is there other assistance you can seek?

4. What are the values relevant to this problem? *Values* are the things that you believe are important in making the decision. They (should) determine priorities. Values relevant to this problem may not be representative of your own personal values or moral framework.

    - Clinic's values: What are the clinic's values?

    - Provider's values: What are the provider's values?

    - Patient: What are the patient's values?

    - Consider compassion, reliability, respect, integrity, trust, commitment, and justice.

5. What are the options for the decision? Think in terms of values and feasibility (e.g., financial, political, organizational, religious constraints).

    - What are the financial costs that should be considered?

    - What are the constraints for political organizations?

    - What are the constraints for religious organizations?

    - What are the consequences of all the potential options?

Management of Case Study

After all considerations, write a short narrative describing the best way to manage this situation; list core values important to you for managing the situation.

Case B: Time Management in Telehealth

This case asks the provider to balance policies and procedures with the need of the patient. This is a common ethical concern in clinical practice and often leads to difficult choices.

Consider:

1. Identify the ethical concerns with this situation.

    - What is the biggest concern for the patient? What are the relevant facts, laws, and principles?

    - What is the biggest concern for the provider? What are the relevant facts, laws, and principles?

2. What information will you need before a responsible decision can be made? (Consider what the information is and where it will come from.)

    - Are there any clinic policies or procedures in place that would help you address this issue/concern?

    - Could there be facts in this case that you are unaware of?

3. Who are the stakeholders involved in the decision, and what is the process in which those involved could come to a decision (e.g., what tools are/could be used to create an informed decision)?

    - Consumer groups: Are there consumer groups that might have input into this issue? What about family or friends?

    - Resources: Are there other resources you could offer the patient?

    - Additional assistance: Is there other assistance you can seek?

4. What are the values relevant to this problem? *Values* are the things that you believe are important in making the decision. They (should) determine priorities. Values relevant to this problem may not be representative of your own personal values or moral framework.

    - What are the clinic's values?

    - What are the provider's values?

    - What are the patient's values?

    - Consider compassion, reliability, respect, integrity, trust, commitment, and justice.

5. What are the options for the decision? Think in terms of values and feasibility (e.g., financial, political, organizational, religious constraints).

    - What are the financial costs that should be considered?

    - What are the constraints for political organizations?

    - What are the constraints for religious organizations?

    - What are the consequences of all the potential options?

Management of Case Study

After all considerations, write a short narrative describing the best way to manage this situation; list core values important to you for managing the situation.

Case C: Pharmaceutical Management Across Prescribing Boundaries

This case explores a common issue in telehealth—managing interstate practice issues. The provider must consider license regulation and other state laws in evaluating the course of action in this dilemma.

Consider:

1. Identify the ethical concerns with this situation.

    - What is the biggest concern for the patient? What are the relevant facts, laws, and principles?

    - What is the biggest concern for the provider? What are the relevant facts, laws, and principles?

2. What information will you need before a responsible decision can be made? (Consider what the information is and where it will come from.)

    - Are there any clinic policies or procedures in place that would help you address this issue/concern?

    - Could there be facts in this case that you are unaware of?

3. Who are the stakeholders involved in the decision, and what is the process in which those involved could come to a decision (e.g., what tools are/could be used to create an informed decision)?

    - Consumer groups: Are there consumer groups that might have input into this particular issue? What about family or friends?

    - Resources: Are there other resources you could offer the patient?

    - Additional assistance: Is there other assistance you can seek?

4. What are the values relevant to this problem? *Values* are the things that you believe are important in making the decision. They (should) determine priorities. Values relevant to this problem may not be representative of your own personal values or moral framework.

    - What are the clinic's values?

    - What are the provider's values?

    - What are the patient's values?

    - Consider compassion, reliability, respect, integrity, trust, commitment, and justice.

5. What are the options for the decision? Think in terms of values and feasibility (e.g., financial, political, organizational, religious constraints).

    - What are the financial costs that should be considered?
    - What are the constraints for political organizations?
    - What are the constraints for religious organizations?
    - What are the consequences of all the potential options?

Management of Case Study

After all considerations, write a short narrative describing the best way to manage this situation; list core values important to you for managing the situation.

CASE STUDY #20

GUIDING A SCHOOL OF NURSING THROUGH COVID-19 FOCUSING ON CLINICAL PLACEMENTS

Leading a school of nursing is a multifaceted and complex assignment in the best of times, rife with decisions potentially impacting generations of nurses. During extraordinary times such as COVID-19, these decisions become more intricate, and the process to make leadership decisions has many potential pitfalls for ethical dilemmas.

Consider:

1. Identify the ethical concerns with this situation.

    - How should the organization, clinical partners, and individuals be considered?

    - What were the costs and benefits of having students in the community-based settings at a time when so much about the virus was unknown? How might this impact future planning?

2. What information will you need before a responsible decision can be made? (Consider what the information is and where it will come from.)

    - Who is directly impacted by these decisions?

    - How would you apply system mapping to visualize how unilateral closure ripples across the system?

    - How would the temporary removal of nursing students from clinical placements impact the other parts of the healthcare system?

3. Who are the stakeholders involved in the decision, and what is the process in which those involved could come to a decision (e.g., what tools are/could be used to create an informed decision)?

    - Which stakeholders would be affected by the temporary removal of nursing students from clinical placements?

    - Consider the needs of federal, state, county, private, and public agencies, and organizations such as the public health department, out-of-hospital healthcare providers, and healthcare point-of-care providers.

4. How would you know if the organizational values are relevant to this problem? *Values* are the things that the organization believes are important in making decisions. Organizational core values should determine priorities.

    - How do you know an organization's values are a fundamental driving force in organizational decisions? Why does sticking to core values require grit?

    - How would the core value of "health for our people, our patients, and our community" impact the decision-making?

5. What are the options for the decision? Think in terms of values and feasibility (e.g., financial, political, organizational, religious constraints).

    - What are considerations for public institutions, private institutions, and not-for-profit health systems' 501-3C status?

    - How does limiting the number of nursing students in clinical placements impact the involved stakeholders, the organization, and the students?

    - Would the course of action decided upon potentially cause others harm? If yes, to whom? If no, why not?

    - What about the potential impact on the nursing workforce if nursing students were delayed in their educational progression?

Management of Case Study

After all considerations, write a short narrative describing the best way to manage this situation; list core values important to you for managing the situation.

CASE STUDY #21

EMERGENCY DEPARTMENT CLOSURE DECISION-MAKING: HEALTH SYSTEM AND COMMUNITY IMPACT

Emergency Medical Services (EMS) are designed to reduce all-cause morbidity and mortality. Emergency departments (EDs) are part of the EMS system. Acute healthcare systems consider diverting inbound patients in periods of overload that saturate facility resources. Diverting EMS transport units has the potential to ripple across the entire EMS system and impact public welfare. Failure to divert incoming patients has the potential to impact healthcare workers and patients already registered and receiving care.

Consider:

1. Identify the ethical concerns with this situation.

    - How should the organization consider the individual person versus the community need for EMS?

    - Discuss ethics of individual rights versus ethics of common good. Ambulance diversion impacts patients who are more reliant on ambulance transportation for healthcare.

2. What information will you need before a responsible decision can be made? (Consider what the information is and where it will come from.)

    - Who should have access to the ED during times of saturation/overcrowding—the patients already in the system or the community at-large?

- How would you apply system mapping to visualize how unilateral closure ripples across the system?
- How would the event of temporary closure impact the other parts of the EMS system?

3. Who are the stakeholders involved in the ambulance diversion plan, and what is the process in which those involved could come to a decision (e.g., what tools are/could be used to create an informed decision)?

    - Federal: What and who are involved at the federal level?
    - State: What and who are involved at the state level?
    - County: What and who are involved at the county level?
    - Private: What and who are involved at the private level?
    - Public agencies and organizations such as the public health department: What are the identified roles of the public organization?
    - Out-of-hospital healthcare provider: What is the role of this provider?
    - Communication systems (911): What needs of the communication system need to be considered?
    - EMS transportation networks (ambulance, air fixed wing, helicopter, national ski patrol): What is the role of the EMS transportation network?
    - Fire department: What is the role of the fire department?
    - First responders (police, paramedics): What tools are provided by first responders?
    - Highly trained healthcare point-of-care providers: What is the role of the healthcare provider?
    - How would you organize a regional working group to establish working relationships among ambulance receiving sites?

4. How would you know if the organizational values are relevant to this problem? *Values* are the things that the organization believes are important in making decisions. Organizational core values should determine priorities.

    - How do you know an organization's values are a fundamental driving force in organizational decisions?
    - Why does sticking to core values require grit?
    - How would the core value of "health for our people, our patients, and our community" impact the decision-making?

5. What are the options for the decision? Think in terms of values and feasibility (e.g., financial, political, organizational, religious constraints).

- Not-for-profit health systems' 501-3C status is based on community benefit. How does limiting community access to the ED impact the organization's community benefit status?

- What is the potential for healthcare policy changes to the Emergency Medical Treatment and Active Labor Act to permit tactical diversion of ambulances?

- How will the organization select the best option for managing saturation?

- Would the course of action decided upon potentially cause others harm?

Management of Case Study

After all considerations, write a short narrative describing the best way to manage this situation; list core values important to you for managing the situation.

CASE STUDY #22

ETHICAL DILEMMAS IN SCHOOL OF NURSING LEADERSHIP PRE-COVID-19

Leadership in schools of nursing in pre-COVID-19 times certainly had unique-to-nursing challenges and ethical dilemmas. Some of those challenges included issues surrounding admissions, student retention, student progression, and student dismissal. Routinely, early in the admissions process, leadership in schools of nursing would feel pressure from institutional sources to admit or give an advantage to one applicant over another due to ties to the institution.

Consider:

1. Identify the ethical concerns with this situation.

   - How should the organization consider the needs of the individual person versus the community members served by nurses?

   - Discuss ethics of individual rights versus ethics of common good. If an executive nurse leader were to pass the student in question, what would be the issues to consider?

   - Behavioral situations are often not clearly black and white due to the difficulties in qualifying and quantifying student behavior. What is the potential impact of a new nurse graduate who exhibits unprofessional behaviors?

   - Who would be impacted and how?

2. What information will you need before a responsible decision can be made? (Consider what the information is and where it will come from.)

   - In addition to student issues, executive leadership are involved with faculty hiring, retention, and promotion in schools of nursing. Ethical concerns in this realm include how to determine who is hired and what rubric is created and applied equitably to minimize subjectivity.

   - What systems are potentially impacted by student and faculty ethical concerns?

   - How would you apply system mapping to visualize the multitude of ripples across the system?

3. Who are the stakeholders involved in the decision, and what is the process in which those involved could come to a decision (e.g., what tools are/could be used to create an informed decision)?

   - Students: What are their roles? How are they affected?

   - Patients: How might patients be affected?

   - Institutions of higher learning: What are their roles in this situation?

   - Future employers of graduates: What is their role?

4. How would you know if the organizational values are relevant to this problem? *Values* are the things that the organization believes are important in making decisions. Organizational core values should determine priorities.

   - How do you know an organization's values are a fundamental driving force in organizational decisions?

   - Why does sticking to core values require grit?

   - How would the core value of "health for our people, our patients, and our community" impact the decision-making?

5. What are the options for the decision? Think in terms of values and feasibility (e.g., financial, political, organizational, religious constraints). Not-for-profit health systems' 501-3C status is based on community benefit.

   - How does passing students with below standard grade point averages or concerning behaviors impact community needs?

   - How will the organization select the best option for managing these situations?

   - Would the course of action decided upon potentially cause others harm?

Management of Case Study

After all considerations, write a short narrative describing the best way to manage this situation; list core values important to you for managing the situation.